YOUR KNOWLEDGE HAS VALUE

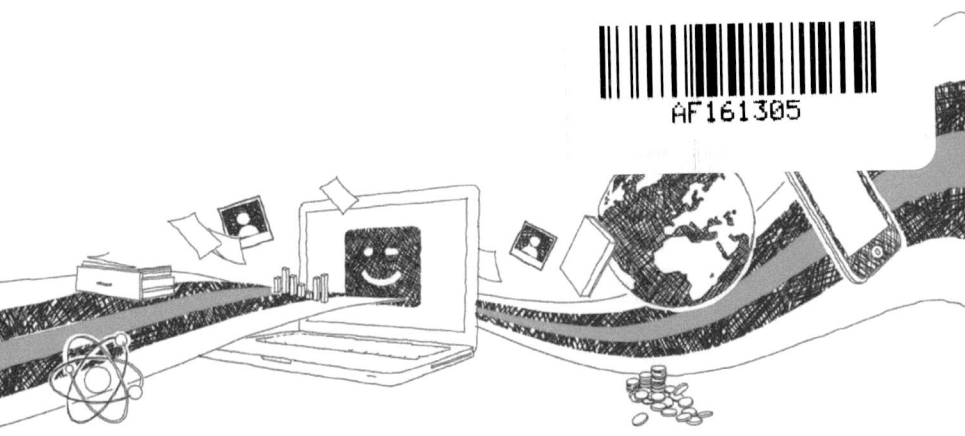

- We will publish your bachelor's and master's thesis, essays and papers

- Your own eBook and book - sold worldwide in all relevant shops

- Earn money with each sale

Upload your text at www.GRIN.com
and publish for free

Bibliographic information published by the German National Library:

The German National Library lists this publication in the National Bibliography; detailed bibliographic data are available on the Internet at http://dnb.dnb.de .

This book is copyright material and must not be copied, reproduced, transferred, distributed, leased, licensed or publicly performed or used in any way except as specifically permitted in writing by the publishers, as allowed under the terms and conditions under which it was purchased or as strictly permitted by applicable copyright law. Any unauthorized distribution or use of this text may be a direct infringement of the author s and publisher s rights and those responsible may be liable in law accordingly.

Imprint:

Copyright © 2015 GRIN Verlag, Open Publishing GmbH
Print and binding: Books on Demand GmbH, Norderstedt Germany
ISBN: 978-3-668-09748-3

This book at GRIN:

http://www.grin.com/en/e-book/311025/gun-policy-a-critical-analysis-of-firearm-laws-in-the-united-states-of

Murali Mg

Gun Policy. A critical analysis of firearm laws in the United States of America

GRIN - Your knowledge has value

Since its foundation in 1998, GRIN has specialized in publishing academic texts by students, college teachers and other academics as e-book and printed book. The website www.grin.com is an ideal platform for presenting term papers, final papers, scientific essays, dissertations and specialist books.

Visit us on the internet:

http://www.grin.com/

http://www.facebook.com/grincom

http://www.twitter.com/grin_com

Contents

Introduction 2

Background Value 3

    History of Gun Violence 4

    Current Gun Laws in the United States of America 8

    The Issue 9

    The Second Amendment 11

United States Gun Laws in contrast with other Countries 12

    Gun Laws in Australia 12

    Gun Laws in India 13

    Gun Law in United Kingdom 13

Bibliography 18

Introduction

The American firearm industry seems to be healthier than ever. The demand and production rates have gone seemingly high and there exist constant demand all over the country for firearm. As per the (Washington times, 2015), during 2013 around 10.8 million of guns were manufactured; which is equivalent to the produced units during 2010 to 2012.

According to the National Vital Statistics, approximately around 31,000 fatalities are recorded each year. The percentage of gun violence or firearm abuse spreads over; suicide (62per cent), homicide (35per cent) and accidental shootings accounts over 3per cent. (Cornell, 2013). Once an individual possess an ownership of a firearm, it makes the job simple and easy; aim and fire. Everyone in the society are vulnerable as the threshold between homicide and anger is brought down (Lendman, 2012).

The mass shooting incident that happened in 2012 which accounted for 26 deaths terrorized the whole United States America. The incident well known remembered as the *Connecticut incident* claimed 20 deaths of school children and six adults has been referred as one of the worst mass shootings in the history of America (Peters, 2013). This is not only the incident that triggered a wide credible debate on the usage of guns and the need for reforms in the existing gun control laws. These facts questions the facets of the current gun laws. "Are the existing gun laws are stricter than ever or weaker than ever?" A report by Centre for American Press, categorized 10 cities that have high rate of gun violence and their study argued that the reason for such high rate of gun violence is due to weaker gun laws (Gerney, Parsons & Posner, 2013). According to Global Research, more people in Chicago are shot and killed than U.S forces in Afghanistan by enemies.

Background Value

According to the U.S Department of Justice, around 68per cent of homicides in America involved guns. In 1996, 34,040 people died from gunfire in the United States. In 2012, around 19,976 suicides were recorded which involved guns. These stats are pretty shocking when compared with the other countries. It doesn't take much time to draw a conclusive analysis about why there are high rates of homicides and suicides that involves firearms and the reason could be argued it because of the flexible Gun laws and policies. A study by (Berkowitz, 1967) argued that the sight of the weapon would trigger aggression from angered persons due to the learned association between weapons and aggressive behavior which makes those angered people exposed to weapons or to any lethal weapons more aggressively. (Kleek, 1988) found out that the deaths that firearms were 3 times higher than the deaths that included knives and other lethal objects.

From the below graph (1), it can be noted that the number of deaths in United States of America is higher than the number of deaths in India, Australia and United Kingdom. It is because in these nations, strong and rigid gun laws are in place. Access to firearms in these countries are forbidden. Even if the citizens wish to possess a firearm, it is not as easy as in United States of America, which is further exposed in this study.

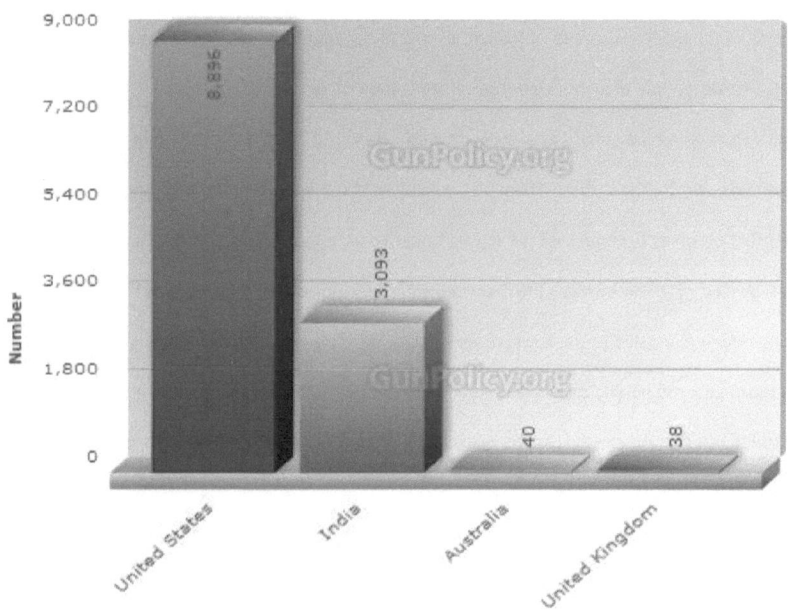

Graph 1: Adapted from Gun Policy, Gun Homicide by Alpers, Philip, Rossetti and Wilson, 2015. Sydney School of Public Health

History of Gun Violence

The history of the gun violence in the United States of America cannot exactly predicted as when it started. According to the conventional theory, the development of the need for possessing firearms began with the English colonists (Deconde, 2001). At that very time, everyone needed guns. Some needed for protection, whilst some needed to carry out illegal activities. The need of possessing a firearm reflects the very essence of positive and negative impact of possessing them. According to the statistics provided by (Gun Violence Archive, 2000), Americans used firearms more often to assault or illegally harm someone, than using them for self-protection during the 20th century. The more disturbing fact is that during 1990's, Americans killed more with guns in week; than the Europeans who used firearms in the whole year (Deconde, 2001). However, there are many incidents where the firearms were used recklessly and irresponsibly killing many human life. The graphical representation presents the annual mass shootings in America, (1982-2012);

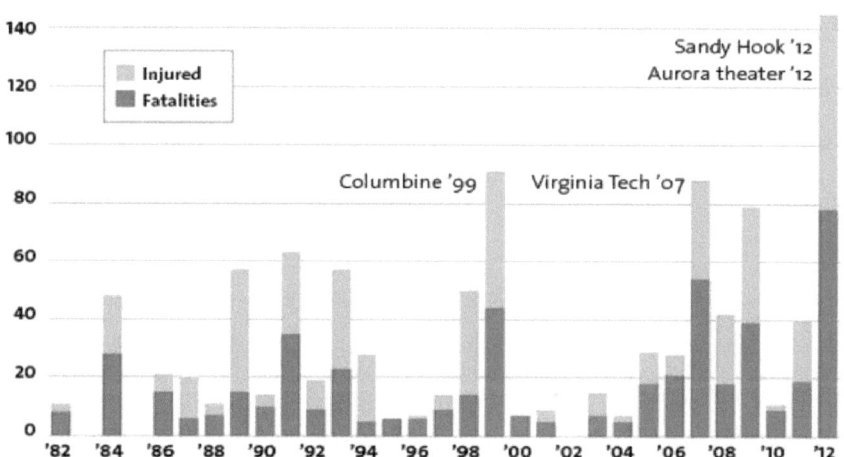

Figure 1:Annual mass shooting casualities. 1982-2012. Mark Follman 2015:

The massacre at the Sandy Hook elementary school (Dec 2012) in Newton is one of those darkest incidents in history of gun violence in America. The incident claimed the lives of 20 children where under the age between 5 to 10 years old and six adults who were horrendously shot down by an armed individual. The incident raised over a nation-wide rage and chaos that confronted the United States of America demanding stricter gun control laws (The Guardian, 2012).

The incident stands out of the other incidents because of the number of deaths tolled and the intensity of a crime. The deaths of 20 young children drew the entire nation into a painful and dark environment."The nihilistic, nature of this intentional, premeditated act; and the characteristics of the victims: young, innocent, defenseless children and the heroic teachers and school staff who died shielding them" (Shultz et al., 2013). The incident was labelled as "fundamentally different" episode of gun violence. It was also described as one of the rarest and extreme event in the history of gun violence.

One of individual who witnessed the incident described the massacre as "the Evil visited our community today". Hundreds of parents ran towards the school to know their children's wellbeing and the agony of the parents who lost their children's was painful (Barron, 2012). In the after math of the incident it was revealed that the 20 year old Adam Lanza, who was responsible for the massacre. He was suffering from personality disorder and was in the need of mental and psychiatric treatment (Faria, 2013).

From Sandy Hook massacre it fairly difficult to debate whether the cause for the shooting was due to ease availability of the guns or obligatory need of development of health care. A study by (Faria 2013) reflected evidences that the cause of such violent shootings is due to the failure of mental health system in the United States of America. One more incident which is referred as the Aurora theatre shooting incident had same intensity as of the Sandy hook massacre. The incident of shooting at Aurora theatre happened on July 20th of 2012. Shortly, after the midnight a gunman opened fire towards the unarmed people who were going to the screening of the movie Batman in the Century 16 theatre complex in Colorado. The incident left 12 dead and more than 82 people were fatally injured.

According to the Action Report, 2014, the gunman fired at least 70 shots towards the crowd; 12 individuals died and 82 people were injured and some them required major surgeries enough to recover. Due to the timely action coordinated between the Aurora city police department, fire emergency and other civil services there were no more fatalities.

The police department of Aurora arrived in less two minutes of the incident coordinating with the rescuers and the emergency ambulance services that reduced the number of furthermore causalities

(Meyer, 2012).The incident absolutely left nothing except nightmare for Aurora and its citizens. In the Century 16th theatre, there was nothing but chaotic environment filled with the dead and wounded lying on the ground trying to move or help the other wounded. The family of the dead or wounded were made wait for days before learning what had happened to their known ones (Denver Post, 2012). Due to the unknown firing there were people running all over the place, which made difficult for the emergency services to get in touch with the wounded. (Denver Post, 2012) "We cannot bypass, there were wounded everywhere and we were unable to get these wounded to others".

The gunmen who opened the fire was identified as 24 year old James Eagan Holmes, who was well equipped with tactical tools was later arrested outside the theatre and was charged with multiple felonies. The culprit later revealed to that he had also placed an explosive equipment in his apartment which was later disarmed with the help of FBI technicians and bomb disbarment teams. The witness who outlined the incident referred it as terrific and chaotic. The culprit used gas bombs to obstruct the vision of the crowd and to cause chaotic environment.

One more incident to highlight in this particular study is the Columbine high school massacre. On April 20th 1999, two teens aged around 18 recklessly opened fire at Columbine high school in Littleton, Colorado killing 13 people and wounding 20 other individuals. The incident video which was recorded on CCTV shows a horrendous visualization of students and other individuals fleeing to save their lives creating havoc and chaos. The video also witnesses the two teens who were on spree on shooting and also an individual who was shot down inside the campus. The petrified students were hiding under the tables and benches to avoid contact with the felonies and to save their lives (Smith, 2012).

The after math of the incident and the investigation revealed that the motive behind the incident was racially biased (History, 2009). The teens who were responsible for the massacre was Harris 17 and Klebold 18, targeted mainly athletes, minorities and Christians as their victims. However, other theories argue that the shootings were carried out in retaliation of being bullied. The teens even shot themselves down committing suicide within the campus only. (Peter 1999), stated that many of the mass shootings including the case of Columbine high school may been because of the cause of rejection, bullied by schoolmates or others. The main cause for the mass shootings within the school environment was due factor that they cannot "fit in" or when students are highly sensitive to teasing and bullying exerts such attitude and behavior, forcing them to carry out such atrocities (Cornell, 1999; Perlstein, 1999).

Current Gun Laws in the United States of America

Laws are subjected to abide the safety and security of the citizens and individuals. The Gun laws in the United States of America differs state to state and are monitored upon by state and federal law.. The rules and laws of possessing a firearm of once city is not applicable to other city. The below Fig (2) outlines the Gun Laws of New York city;

	RIFLES & SHOTGUNS	HANDGUNS
Permit to Purchase	No*	Yes
Registration of Firearms	No*	Yes
Licensing of Owners	No*	Yes
Permit to Carry	No*	Yes

Figure 2: Adapted from Gun Laws, NRA-ILA.2012

According to NRA-ILA

- **SHALL ISSUE** State Law that provides that upon, completion of specific requirements, a law-abiding person shall be granted a permit to carry concealed firearms.
- **DISCRETIONARY/REASONABLE ISSUE** State law that provides the government with some discretion over the issuance of a carry permit, but which generally grants permits to all law-abiding persons.

- **NO PERMIT REQUIRED** State law that allows individuals to carry concealed firearms for lawful purposes without a permit.
- **RIGHTS RESTRICTED - VERY LIMITED ISSUE** State law that gives the government complete discretion over the issuance of carry permits, and where that discretion is normally used to deny the issuance of permits.
- **RIGHTS INFRINGED/NON-ISSUE** State law that completely prohibits carrying firearms for personal protection outside the home or place of business.
- **According to the Second Amendment,** A well regarded militia, being necessary to the security of free-state, the right of people to keep and bear arms, shall not be infringed.

According to the Federal Gun Control Act of 1968, under U.S.C 922, the sale of firearms are prohibited to any individual if they are; *underage, fugitive from justice, convicted, or is under indictment, a crime punishable by imprisonment for more than a year, unlawful user or addicted to a controlled substance, mentally defective, committed to a mental institution, is an illegal alien, dishonorably discharged from military service, renounced U.S. Citizenship, convicted of misdemeanor offense of domestic violence.*

The Issue

According to (Gun Policy, 2014), the estimated number of total civilians possessing different firearms in the United States of America accounted for about 270,000,000 to 310,000,000 which is literally one of the shocking facts to believe. Another stats reveal that the estimated rate of private gun ownership in the United States is 101.05 firearms per 100 people and during 2012 around 8,896 deaths were totaled as firearms homicide.

Lastly, United States of America stands No.1 in the list of countries who have private ownership of possessing firearms. The availability of firearms within the ease is the one factor that can argued and noted as a possible factors that cause for violence and crime. The above stats reveals that how it is easy to possess a firearm in the United States of America. One of the major loophole in the gun laws is that the when a buyer privately purchase a firearm, he/she need not to provide any identity for background checks. According to the current law, while buying a firearm the background checks on the buyer can be delayed for a period time or it need not to be done. This gives an easy access to individuals to possess firearms. In most of the cities of United States of America, an individual need not possess a permit to carry a firearm (NRA-ILA). According to Law Centre to Prevent Gun Violence, around 67,000 firearms were listed to sale online by private and unlicensed sellers. Such sellers provide ease of access to firearms to individuals.

It is not that the all individuals who possess a firearm are criminals or they might use it for violence or assaulting someone, it is the notion that if everyone or majority of them possess a firearm there exist a considerable danger. However, by performing background checks before issuing the ownership over a firearm, could possibly result in decline of such violence.

Contradictorily, such a check cannot be done as there exist various variations and factors. It is not only about gun violence, but also about the suicides used with firearms. It quite becomes difficult to monitor or perform a check on individuals. However, background checks might help in reduce the sale of firearms to felons and criminals. The ownership for possessing a firearm should be made more rigid. Firearms shouldn't be a piece of candy that can be purchased in any retail store. It is a harmful and assault device that can fatal any human and it should be sold with effective precautions and measures. The sale of large capacity of firearms or ammunition should be restricted.

The sale of any firearm to any individual should be linked to their personality profiles so that it shall be easy to monitor. According to (Gutterman, 2015) states with most gun deaths have high gun ownership. Alaska is one among the cities that has highest gun ownerships has resulted in most of the firearm fatalities. A strong gun laws such as like New York, had resulted low number of fatalities caused by firearms. There should be more rigid rules on the licensed sellers. A survey of state prison, outlined the fact the majority of gun offenders and murderers obtained the firearms from a gun store or pawnshop where backgrounds are required. These demands the need of stricter background checks. A federal background check could limit the sale of firearms to offenders which would likely to reduce gun violence in the nation and such a system should be extended to the whole of the nation. Some of the main areas improvement on current gun laws is briefed below;

- Background checks on the buyer at the point of sales.
- Ban of sale of large firearms and ammunition and ban on sale of firearms to convicts.
- Restricting the sale firearms other than handgun or pistols for private buyers.
- Constantly reviewing and renewing the license of the owners.
- Ban on sale of firearms to individuals under the age 25 years.

The Second Amendment

According to the second amendment, "A well-regulated militia, being necessary to the security of a free state, the right of people to keep and bear arms, shall not be infringed. Such act is technically naïve. It suggests that people can possess any sort arms and ammunition if they possess an ability and skills. That means an individual with an ability can possess a machine gun or a military tank or highly-skilled weapons that could seriously damage that would result in mass destruction. Even this move, is completely dishonored by the pro-gunners.

However, the act even states it should be a regulated militia and it doesn't cover an average citizen and there will be no serious damage to any average citizen (Sixth Court, 1971). However, even a person with suitable skills and abilities, he/she is living within the country and not in the warzone, such rule or act cannot be imposed within country or state or city; a unstable militia may open a fire in an open and can cause serious damage using sophisticated weapons. Instead, the government should provide with police and security personnel's with more training and additional weapons kit; For instance providing the local Police Departments with an elite weapons would be an advantage in tackling some unfavorable scenarios, rather than vesting sophisticated weapons in the hands of citizen. To conclude, to reduce the fatalities caused by firearms, stricter gun laws are required and the main focus should be kept on ownership, permit, background checks and personality profiles. There should also be a team in each state to evaluate an applicant's need before issuing any sorts of the firearm.

United States Gun Laws in contrast with other Countries

Gun Laws in Australia

Gun laws in Australia were once flexible as in like United States of America, however gun laws underwent certain changes and amendments over duo course of time. According to Firearms Act 1996, an adult may apply for the license by providing the evidence that the applicant' identity with accordance to the requirements under the Financial Transaction Reports Act 1988, that apply in relation to the opening of bank account, and contain information prescribed by regulation, and be accompanied by the document prescribed by regulation (Australian Capital Territory, 2015). During the application process the registrar informs the applicant to go through certain training program. The registrar may the applicant to provide any further documents and he/she may request to disclose the mental health record at any point of the application process. The Australian Government is pretty much strict about their gun laws.

Primarily, an adult cannot possess a gun without a license as it would be illegal; he/she has to fill an application enclosed with authenticate documents which serves as an identity and would be helpful in background checks. After a mass shooting massacre in 1996 in Australia that left 35 dead, the government came hard on the existing gun laws and forced stricter laws by completing banning the ownership of semi-automatic and shot rifles for citizens. The Australian government provided a scheme "buyback scheme" where the citizens of Australia surrendered their weapons. This move changed the rates of mass shootings and homicides. After making amendments to Gun Laws, there were no single case reported about shootings or homicides in Australia. According to the research of (Leigh and Neil, 2012), firearm homicide rate by 59per cent and the firearm suicide fell by 65per cent. A study by (Chapman, Alpers, Agho and Jones, 2006) presented empirical evidences that proved there was no single incidence of mass shooting, since the revision of existing gun laws.

Gun Laws in India

In India the gun laws are regulated and monitored by The Arms Act, 1959. According to the Arms Act 1959, no individual should acquire, have in his possession or carry any firearm or ammunition unless he holds the behalf a license issues in accordance to The ARMS ACT 1959 (Ministry of Affairs). Indian gun laws are very rigid when compared to Australia. In India no citizen is authorized to possess a gun in his/her ownership.

Gun Law in United Kingdom

In United Kingdom too, firearms policies are pretty rigid. In UK firearms are considered too dangerous and lethal weapons and the state has duty to protect the public from their misuse and owning a gun in United Kingdom is a privilege and not an exercised right. A individual can avail a ownership of firearm will be given, only when an individual is assessed by the licensing authority, the police and that he/she should be posing a potential threat and should have genuine reason for owning a firearm. Individuals who have been convicts for more than 3 years cannot obtain an ownership of a firearm or an ammunition. Before giving a license to avail a firearm, there shall be number of checks and which includes person's property, criminal records, checks and references from friends (Home Office, 2015). The number of guns in the United Kingdom is 11,227 only.

According to the analysis, in India and United Kingdom, it is pretty impossible to buy firearms and will not be considered as threat to the country. Australia once had flexible gun laws, however due to the increase in mass shooting; the government of Australia decided to induce stricter laws for Gun control. In 2011, the United Kingdom had 0.07 gun homicides for every 100,000 people, whilst the United States had 3 gun homicides for every 100,000 people; this outlines the stricter gun laws that are present in the United Kingdom. In United Kingdom, usage of semi-automatic rifles, machine guns, pump action rifles, manually loaded cartridge and pistols are completely banned and prohibited as according to the English rifle and gun club legal center. Prior to 1996, Australia had 15 guns for every 100 people and high number of shootings were recorded. However, the attempt by Pro-gun conservative John Howard pushed through an effective and ambitious gun program, which was also accepted by the citizens of Australia that banned all automatic and semi-automatic guns and also increased the background checks and extended waiting purchase periods (Hickey, 2013).

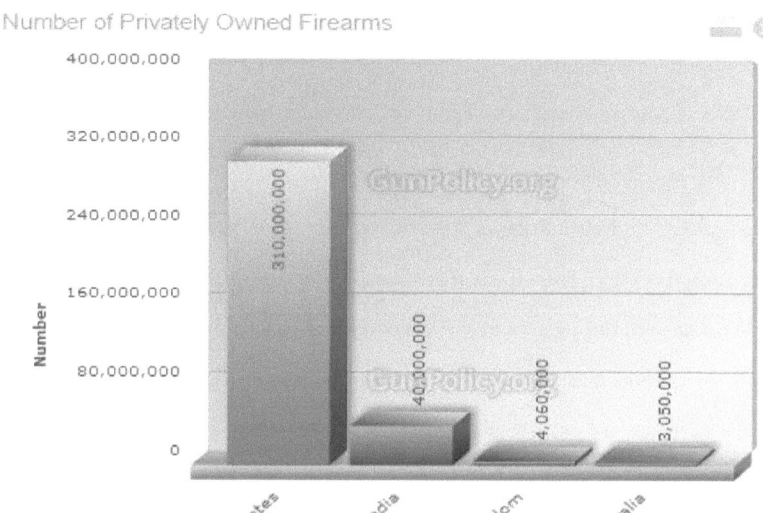

Graph 2: Adapted from Gun Policy, Guns in Australia by Alpers, Philip, Wilso & Rosetti, 2015, Syndney School of Public Health.

The above chart represents the number of privately owned firearms by four nations; United States of America, India, United Kingdom and Australia. The graph represents all. India, having more than 1 billion population has around 40 million individual possessing firearms, which is more likely to be on specific job reason and purpose. In contrast with United Kingdom and Australia, the numbers who are possessing firearms are seemingly less; which represents the nations greater importance laid security of the citizens and strong gun laws that are in place.

Whilst in United Kingdom and Australia, it's a complete different picture, according to stats they have around 4,060,000 and 3,050,000 privately owned firearms which seemingly low that India itself. In contrast with United States of America, the possession of firearms in the country is very high and its staggering growth rate is highly questionable and fearsome. What would happen if number of private ownership of firearms keeps growing and everyone possess a firearm. Henceforth, it is suggested that the United States of America should consider to regulate stricter gun laws to secure the citizens of America.

In this paper gun laws in United States of America has critically reflected under different varying variables. Of course, the United States is one of best and top sovereign country and a nation of freedom where people has an exclusive right exercise their constitutional and voices. However, keeping Gun Laws flexibly would create more chaos rather a secured environment. The mass shooting in United States is now not common and the firearm homicide and suicide rates are clinging. It is not suggested that the United States should ban entire usage of Guns and firearms in the nation, but it is advised to regulate rigid gun laws, so firearms aren't purchased as toys from the retail store. These equipment, machineries and lethal weapons which can cause serious threat and injury to any individual. So keeping it in the mind, the government has improvise the standard procedures before issuing firearm license. It should learn the laws that have been placed in neighboring countries.

Background checks should strengthened, no should be allowed to buy a firearm instantly, ban on automatic and semi-automatic should be enforced upon. Training procedures should be enhanced and a separate counselling sessions should be arranged before issuing the ownership for possessing a firearm.

To conclude, apparently it is true; Gun Laws should protect people and not the opposite. Not everyone needs a firearm to protect themselves, citizens should not buy a firearm for purpose fancy. The government has strengthen law and order to ensure maximum security is provided to their citizens which eventually reduces the number of people incidents to use a firearm. In a nation like United States, metal detectors should be place in each and every school, colleges, civil service offices, hospitals and in other places where large crowds are expected. Finally, the existing gun laws do have loopholes, however, each law and rules have loopholes and people with bad intentions and unstable conditions exploit them to harm the citizens. Henceforth, to avoid such violent incident, the government of United States of America should think about it and regulate the rules of existing gun laws to permanently close those loop holes.

Bibliography

ACT Parliamentary Counsel, (2015). *Firearms Act 1996* (pp. 6-18). Australia: ACT Parliamentary Counsel.

Alpers, P. (2015). *Gun Law and Policy: Firearms and armed violence, country by country. Gunpolicy.org*. Retrieved 6 April 2015, from http://www.gunpolicy.org/

Business Insider,. (2015). *How Australia And Other Developed Nations Have Put A Stop To Gun Violence*. Retrieved 3 April 2015, from http://www.businessinsider.in/How-Australia-And-Other-Developed-Nations-Have-Put-A-Stop-To-Gun-Violence/articleshow/21447576.cms

Center for American Press,. (2013). *America Under the Gun: A 50 state analysis of Gun Violence and its link to weak state gun laws* (pp. 9-17). Washington D C: American Press.

Chapman, S., Alpers, P., Agho, K., & Jones, M. (2006). Australia's 1996 gun law reforms: faster falls in firearm deaths, firearm suicides, and a decade without mass shootings. *Injury Prevention*, *12*(6), 365-372. doi:10.1136/ip.2006.013714

Cheng, X. (2002). *Analysis of states of gun control restrictions* (Master's in Art). University of South Florida.

DeConde, A. (2001). *Gun violence in America*. Boston: Northeastern University Press.

Denverpost.com,. (2015). *Aurora to get analysis of theater shooting response*. Retrieved 28 March 2015, from http://www.denverpost.com/news/ci_25478749/aurora-get-analysis-theater-shooting-response

Faria, M. (2013). Shooting rampages, mental health, and the sensationalization of violence. *Surg Neurol Int*, *4*(1), 16. doi:10.4103/2152-7806.106578

Gabbatt, A., & Williams, M. (2012). *Newtown gunman kills 20 children in elementary school shooting*. *The Guardian*. Retrieved 1 April 2015, from http://www.theguardian.com/world/2012/dec/14/newtown-shooting-gunman-kills-20-children

Global Research,. (2015). *Gun Violence in America*. Retrieved 2 April 2015, from http://www.globalresearch.ca/gun-violence-in-america/5315892

http://www.apa.org,. (2015). *Gun Violence: Prediction, Prevention, and Policy*. Retrieved 3 April 2015, from http://www.apa.org/pubs/info/reports/gun-violence-prevention.aspx

Law Center to Prevent Gun Violence,. (2015). *LAWS & POLICIES*. Retrieved 6 April 2015, from http://smartgunlaws.org/gun-policy/

Leigh, A., & Neill, C. (2010). Do Gun Buybacks Save Lives? Evidence from Panel Data. *American Law And Economics Review*, *12*(2), 509-557. doi:10.1093/aler/ahq013

More Guns, Less Crime: Understanding Crime and Gun Control laws. (2010) (3rd ed., pp. 37-68). Liberty of Congress-Pub.

NPR.org,. (2013). *Rate Of U.S. Gun Violence Has Fallen Since 1993, Study Says*. Retrieved 5 April 2015, from http://www.npr.org/blogs/thetwo-way/2013/05/07/181998015/rate-of-u-s-gun-violence-has-fallen-since-1993-study-says

Nraila.org,. (2015). Retrieved 30 March 2015, from https://www.nraila.org

Peters, R. (2013). *When will the US learn from Australia? Stricter gun control laws save lives | Rebecca Peters*. *the Guardian*. Retrieved 6 April 2015, from http://www.theguardian.com/commentisfree/2013/dec/14/america-mass-murder-australia-gun-control-saves-lives

Planning Corporation, T. (2014). *Aurora Century 16 Theater Shooting* (pp. 38-57). Aurora.

Rt.com,. (2015). *22 million Americans have anger issues & own a gun – study*. Retrieved 2 April 2015, from http://rt.com/usa/248377-americans-anger-gun-ownership/

Shultz, J., Cohen, A., Muschert, G., & Flores de Apodaca, R. (2013). Fatal school shootings and the epidemiological context of firearm mortality in the United States. *Disaster Health*, *1*(2), 84-101. doi:10.4161/dish.26897

Shultz, J., Muschert, G., Dingwall, A., & Cohen, A. (2013). The Sandy Hook Elementary School shooting as tipping point. *Disaster Health*, *1*(2), 65-73. doi:10.4161/dish.27113

The Huffington Post,. (2015). *States With Most Gun Deaths Have High Gun Ownership And Weaker Gun Laws, Report Shows*. Retrieved 1 April 2015, from http://www.huffingtonpost.com/2015/01/29/weak-gun-laws-and-high-gu_n_6572384.html?ir=India

Webster, D., & Vernick, J. (2014). *Updated evidence and policy developments on reducing gun violence in America*. Baltimore, Md.: Johns Hopkins University Press.

Wright, J., Rossi, P., Daly, K., & Weber, E. (1983). *Under the gun*. New York: Aldine Pub. Co.

YOUR KNOWLEDGE HAS VALUE

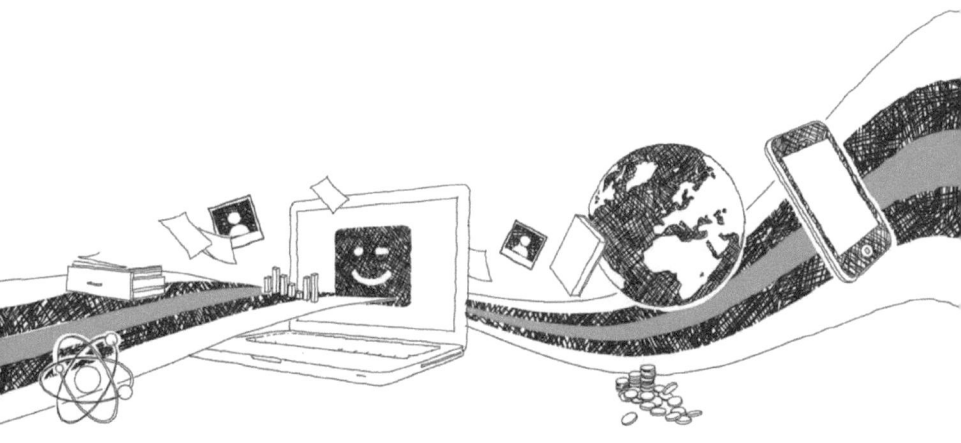

- We will publish your bachelor's and master's thesis, essays and papers

- Your own eBook and book - sold worldwide in all relevant shops

- Earn money with each sale

Upload your text at www.GRIN.com
and publish for free

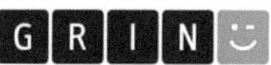